Russian Clay Secrets

Medicinal and Cosmetic
Applications of Healing Clay

By Matt Isaac

Russian Clay Secrets: Medicinal and
Cosmetic Applications of Healing Clay

By Matt Isaac

ISBN: 978-0-9836339-0-7

Questions, comments:
http://www.russianclaytherapy.info

Published by Bread Line Publishing
Printed in the USA
Design & Layout by EditWriteDesign.com

Disclaimer: The purpose of this work is to provide as accurate
information as possible regarding the subject of clay therapy.
The actions and ideas put forth in this book are not intended
to replace a consultation with a physician or other medical
specialists. The author and/or publisher are not engaged in
any professional medical services and are not liable for any
injury, loss, or other damages purportedly caused by the use
of the information found in this book.

Acknowledgement

For my Grandparents

Contents

4. Specific Green Clay Treatments   27

5. Cosmetic Applications w/Green Clay   61

6. Different Colored Clay   73

Bibliography   95

About the Author   97

1

Introduction

"This vast ball, the Earth, was molded out of clay, and baked in fire." **- Henry Wadsworth Longfellow (1807-1882)**

Clay is embedded in our lives

Since the beginning, clay has nurtured our development as a species. Through all this time until today clay has remained in our lives. Therefore, it is a mistake to look at clay therapy as a new method or a passing fad that has entered into our lives only to leave in a few short years or even months. And it is even a bigger mistake to look at clay as an outdated remedy.

You can even open the Bible and notice the importance of clay:

> *"Therefore said they unto him, How were thine eyes opened? He answered and said, A man that is called Jesus made clay, and anointed mine eyes, and said unto me, Go to the pool of Siloam, and wash: and I went and washed, and I received sight." John 9:10*

1

It is possible that, in this particular passage, the Bible alludes to the healing properties of red clay found on the banks of the Nile. Although during those early days people didn't study clay's medicinal properties, they had already discovered its "magical" power.

Today, the great properties of the Nile's clay are well-known, as well as how Egyptians benefited from it for hundreds of years. In addition to making pots, clay powder was mixed with tobacco and other plants to create healing balms, which were used for their antiseptic and haemostatic (*the process that causes bleeding to stop*) properties and to accelerate the healing process.

Clay has always drawn attention from people and for a long time remained the main method of healing. Pliny the Elder and Avicenna oftentimes recommended adding clay to medicinal herbs—something that herbalists still do today—to amplify the curing properties of the mixture as a whole and decrease the necessary duration of treatments. Until this day, their medical advice is still relevant and extremely valuable.

Clay was deeply rooted in Roman body care. In his great work, *Naturalis Historia*, Pliny the Elder wrote about a clay possessing a greenish color. He mentioned how the Romans added this clay to their baths along with mineral water that they acquired from the mountains of Italy. People prepared mud baths with varied consistency to clean and soften their skin. Clay was also widely accepted for its abilities to make skin smooth in places where there were dry and rough patches.

Pliny the Elder further pointed out that clay plays a stabilizing role in our organisms. Ancient Romans were well aware of the anti-inflammatory and antiseptic properties of clay as they regularly added it to painful areas of the body and deep wounds. Clay was used not only to treat people, but animals as well; thick and heavy layers of clay were used to cover horses' wounds so that they would heal faster.

Until the 18th Century, pharmacists had an in-depth knowledge of clay's therapeutic properties, as well as how to properly prepare it for external and internal medicinal use. As medicine advanced, though, clay was quickly forgotten. It was only during World War I (1914-1918), when it became nearly impossible to find any medicine in France, that people remembered about clay. In the absence of hygiene and proper nutrition, both the French and the Russians used clay to prevent and treat dysentery (*an inflammatory disorder of the lower intestinal tract, usually caused by a bacterial, parasitic, or protozoan infection and resulting in pain, fever, and severe diarrhea, often accompanied by the passage of blood and mucus*), an ailment which often proved to be fatal if left untreated.

Clay in Russia

In the first part of the 1900's, as the United States was bursting into the Chemical Age, Russia was being held back by wars: World War I in 1914, the Russian Revolution in 1917, followed by World War II. Unlike the United States, which was able to use these wars for profit and technological advancements, Russia was left devastated. And although Russia was able to eventually climb to a military superpower status after WWII, its culture and industry fell far behind its main competitor, the United States.

A lagging industrial production, along with communist politics, forced the people of Russia to live mainly off the land. To survive, the majority had to know not only how to farm, but how to use the Earth for its healing powers as well.

Even after technology and science began to advance, Russians remained closer than ever to nature and its wonderful gifts. To this day, although there is a growing trend in the United States of people going back to natural healing alternatives, Russia still finds itself as the center of advanced natural medicine.

In this book, I have pulled together information from interviews, websites, modern literature, and businesses in Russia that revolve around clay therapy in order to provide you with healing recipes and cosmetic treatments that are currently in use. The information mostly belongs to the Russian people who stand behind clay therapy and have been practicing their trade for the last few decades, intertwining their natural healing knowledge with modern scientific information to produce phenomenal results.

Yet with so much information at my fingertips, I still had to decide which bits and pieces would be the most beneficial to the reader. There have been some great books published recently that have really well-laid out information on different types of clay and how they work. Although this book starts with some overview, it is very brief and general because it has a slightly different focus: to give a clay lover some addition application methods with a different cultural perspective.

Clay today

There are people who turn to clay as a source of nutrition. Anthropologists have confirmed that primitive people were able to survive for months, and even years, by consuming clay dissolved in water and mixed with plant roots. It has been documented that even with this seemingly poor diet, people did not experience a significant nutritional deficiency. In India and Africa, it is still common today to swallow a few pieces of clay with every meal.

Some nations, attributing a magical power to clay, believe that it expels evil spirits. During certain phases of the moon, native tribes cover themselves in clay to get rid of disease-causing curses. A ceremony is scheduled strictly according to the lunar calendar and is meticulously performed to reinforce the belief that clay can cleanse a soul of all evils.

Scientific research and recent developments in technology and biotechnology have opened new horizons for clay in developed countries as well. Studies have revealed clay's structure, composition, physiochemical properties, etc., and opened up new doors for its use.

Raw clay material is already used in many industries that manufacture hygienic and cosmetic products. It is also regularly added as an anti-allergy component in a variety of new synthetic products on the market, since many of the new synthetics cause allergic reactions.

Recent research and publications of centuries-old applications of clay have made it difficult for today's doctors to dismiss the benefits. Today, we are seeing the use of clay spreading day by day and showing the most significant growth in developed countries. One of the main reasons this is happening is that clay's role as a preventive measure and treatment in many ways is still superior to the synthetic approach of the drug companies. It also helps that more and more people today are demanding highly-effective medications that are developed through natural means without any uncomfortable or harmful side effects.

Regardless of the form of presentation—capsules, bags, tablets, powder, and powder mixed with other medical products—clay continues to play a leading role as an alternative healing method. Some even view it as a panacea for all ailments and flock to health food stores to buy it.

Yet, despite the numerous and revealing scientific studies, clay's secrets are not fully uncovered, and some properties of clay still remain unexplained. Unsatisfied with only a partial explanation a big part of the medical community still attempts to suppress clay from modern medical practice; however, the nearing revelation of clay's ultimate secrets could be the discovery of the century.

2

Clay Specifics

"You cannot help but learn more as you take the world into your hands. Take it up reverently, for it is an old piece of clay, with millions of thumbprints on it." **- John Updike (1932-2009)**

Clay is elastic, soft, and fragile; easily scratched (*method for determining hardness*); during hard impact, it forms cracks; it easily crumbles when dry. In high temperatures clay loses its elasticity and the ability to absorb liquid. In its crushed form, it is used as a component in the ceramic industry, where it does not lose its shape when heated.

Certain types of clay, including illite, consist of over 40 minerals. The main ones are: oxygen (O), silicon (Si), calcium (Ca), aluminum (A1), magnesium (Mg), iron (Fe), cobalt (Co), manganese (Mn), and potassium (K). Other elements, including lithium, copper, and molybdenum are present in extremely small amounts; however, even those small amounts play an important role in aiding cells' daily functions.

Elements possess electromagnetic properties. The electric charge of the particles—positive and negative—creates a force. They are either drawn towards each other or push each other away, creating an electromagnetic field. It is due to these magnetic properties that clay is able to capture and retain foreign elements within its structure. In much the same way, clay can absorb exudates (*fluid oozing in the area of an inflammation*), and thus clean tissues of an ailing organism.

Silicon

Silicon is the basic component of all living tissues alongside magnesium, calcium, and phosphorus. It interacts with magnesium and calcium to help our organisms absorb vitamin D.

On this basis, silicon is considered extremely important in delaying the processes of aging as well as being a preventive measure against cancer. It regenerates skin cells and is great for anyone at any age, but especially the elderly. Older generations can also benefit from silicon because it slows the loss of calcium, which is usually responsible for the development of bone diseases at an older age.

It is difficult to overestimate the importance of silicon during a fight with an infectious disease as it activates the development of antibodies by raising the organism's resistance and suppressing the spread of disease-causing microbes.

Aluminum

Aluminum stabilizes various functions of a living organism. However, aluminum can only be consumed in tiny doses. The small percentage contained in green clay is just the right amount and is quite sufficient to reduce stress.

You can also take aluminum when you have trouble falling asleep or if you are feeling restless.

Calcium

Calcium is essential for any living organism, particularly for cell functions. It regulates digestive systems, helps to create new blood cells, and interacts with phosphorous in restoring bones.

Bone fibers have a high percentage of calcium. And although it seems that bones are not chemically reacting with blood, scientific research has proven that there is a constant ionic exchange between the two. A shortage of calcium in an organism may lead to the following diseases:

- Osteitis (*inflammation of the bones*) - an infringement on the regenerative function of cells in a bone, oftentimes resulting in irreversible bone deformations.

- Osteomalacia (*softening of the bones*) - caused by a lack of calcium and phosphorous. As time goes on, bones become increasingly frail.

- Osteoporosis (*lowering bone mineral density*) - which leads to an increased risk of bone fracture.

- Rickets and spasmophilia may also develop when there is a lack of calcium.

Absorption

A key characteristic of clay that makes it so great for medical and cosmetic use is absorption. It is easier to explain this property if you think of clay as a sponge. In much the same way, clay absorbs water and slightly expands.

The difference, however, is that while absorbing elements from the water, clay shares its elements with the water as well. The exchange continues until equilibrium is reached. Hence, when clay comes in contact with skin, internal organs, or even with the ground, the process is similar.

All types of clay have the ability to absorb water; nevertheless, the various types have their own characteristics that make them different from one another.

For example, the top surface of illite clay, for example, has a high electric charge that permits the water to flow through quite quickly; this flow allows for instant reactions and establishes favorable conditions for ionic exchange. (As clay expands, the hydration process slows down. Consequently, the ionic exchange slows down.)

Adsorption

Adsorption, an accumulation of particles on the surface, is also a key characteristic of clay that makes it so great for medical and cosmetic use. It is a physiochemical property of clay that causes things—toxins, microbes, waste—to stick to the outside surface. Between the plates of clay there are small spaces which remain even during the process of absorption. These spaces become filled with gases as well as pathogenic (*capable of causing disease*) microbes. In this way clay can be used to draw in the toxins. This explains clay's sensitivity to its surrounding environment as well as why it is extremely useful to us. As clay adsorbs the toxins and pulls it away from the organism, the organism can regain its strength and get back to a healthy state once again.

Illite

When you go to the store that carries green clay, it is possible that the packaging will indicate that it is an illite clay. This type of clay comes from northern parts of the world that was once covered by sea. During the formation, sea minerals of glacial origin were constantly bombarded with rain, wind, and layers of ground stacking one on top of the other over time. The basic makeup of this clay is 70-80% illite, 5-10% kaolinite, and about as much of montmorillonite. Such a complex mineral structure partly explains why this clay can be so useful.

Illite is extracted from mines where it lies in layers kind of like big pieces of butter. The pieces extracted usually measure around 10 yards in length and width and are lifted from depths of more than 200 feet. Each year hundreds of tons of this clay are extracted to meet our daily needs.

Montmorillonite

Montmorillonite usually has a pale gray-green color. It is often known as "green clay." This swelling clay is widely used in medicine and pharmacology. The chemical makeup is very close to that of illite, but the formation of minerals is very different.

Montmorillonite has a very high absorbency and can hold eight times its own volume in liquid. It is viscous, sticky, and has a difficulty maintaining a shape. It is often used in the food industry, in particular, to degrease and filter wine and champagne.

Bentonite

Bentonite, sometimes called montmorillonite because it is the main make of this type of clay, is able to absorb water many times its own volume.

The slowed down process of hydration is the reason why this clay is extremely sticky and viscous. It is also a contributing factor to the useful properties of the unstable electromagnetic field of the clay.

A few common uses of bentonite:

- Wine filtration

- Building bridges (as a component of cement)

- As a binding agent in manufacturing paints

- To make the sticky coating in nail polish

Sun, water and clay

Broadly speaking, there is no life without the sun. And among its many gifts, the sun plays a role of a cleanser here on Earth. As an organic source of heat, the sun naturally dries clay, while killing microbes inside it, and thus cleaning the clay without harming the nutrients within.

Like clay, water has a complex structure, often consisting of many more elements than we might initially suspect. Water naturally strengthens specific properties of clay by separating and activating the elements within the clay structure. In simplified terms, water serves as a transportation device for ions. Without water these ions would not be able to penetrate into the tiniest places in our bodies.

The charged particles, optimized by solar energy, are able to get free thanks to passing water ions. Once free, they can strengthen the physiochemistry of the surrounding environment and stabilize the magnetic field of the clay's minerals.

<u>REMEMBER</u>

CLAY WITHOUT WATER
IS CLAY WITHOUT LIFE!

Preservation and quality control

The quality control procedures for clay have been developed into a meticulous process. In all three stages—before storing, while packaging and after it is on the shelves—clay is tested for quality; measured for mineral consistency; undergoes microbiological analysis; and physical and chemical tests are done as well. This type of rigorous testing allows a company to guarantee its customers good quality clay.

Under the current European norms, the rules that apply to storing clay are the same ones that apply to storing food. Therefore, before clay goes on sale—during extraction, production, and final manufacturing phases—it is put to numerous microbiological tests.

Some of the test results are displayed on the package, which should at least indicate the mineral makeup of the clay along with the physiochemical properties to allow the customer to determine the quality of the product and its ability to help during a confrontation with a disease or a cosmetic issue.

Natural clay, which can be found in many stores, shows all the key information that a customer needs to check for quality. For example, it should indicate that the clay was never exposed to any preservatives during the drying and storage periods.

Clay itself has to meet specific requirements as well. It should have been heated up and dried on the sun to neutralize the dense microflora. This approach leads to complete loss of water and certain unnecessary elements.

If in doubt, call the manufacturer. Have the necessary information to describe the product and the expiration date. They should provide you with the results of the microbiological testing conducted on your specific clay. (For your health's sake, you should not forgo this little bit of extra research on your part.)

Although most manufacturers are going through all the meticulous steps of delivering a safe and an effective product, you should always act with caution, as the quality of a product always depends on its content. Make sure you know it well!

How to choose your clay

Not all clays work equally well for therapeutic purposes. You should learn to choose the right one for you. To make the right selection, consider the following properties of green clay:

- It should not contain large grains, which you can feel scratch along your teeth when you make a clay shake.

- When prepared, it should shine and have a homogeneous dough-like consistency.

- The packaging should indicate the minerals and elements that are contained in the clay.

- When clay is dry, it should have a light green color.

- When wet, it should have a dark green color.

- Also make sure that the packaging indicates that it is safe to ingest.

- Another sign of quality is when the package indicates that the clay has been sun dried.

- The highest quality clay is illite green clay. It has been sold in some stores for over fifty years. Illite clay can typically be applied externally and internally and in the form of a compress. (It is also used as a food additive.)

3

Preparing Green Clay Treatments

"I have but shadowed forth my intense longing to lose myself in the Eternal and become merely a lump of clay in the Potter's divine hands so that my service may become more certain because uninterrupted by the baser self in me." **- Mohandas Gandhi**

The elements present in green clay ultimately strengthen the immune function of an organism. The immune system is then better able to fight diseases and promote the restoration and stabilization of intracellular exchange, which occurs continuously, millions of times over, in our organisms. Those elements also play an integral role as a prophylactic against infectious diseases. And they further help in the regeneration process while establishing a harmony among the many processes within a living cell.

The best time to use clay

Treatment is best suited for spring and autumn. In the spring, during the first signs of nature waking, we immediately have a deep desire, even if hidden, to bare ourselves to the world and to do so with a fresh and energetic look. We can attain this look by removing all the waste that has collected in our bodies over the winter. This will require daily work and attention for a period of time.

Green clay contains the necessary elements to assist with all the functions of an organism. By properly using green clay, your body will receive the right mixture of elements to aid those functions. Like the snow melting under the warm rays of the sun, green clay can remove the accumulated toxins from your body.

On the other hand, applying green clay during the fall will prepare your body for the upcoming short days, when the sun hovers slightly over the horizon and our bodies decrease in activity and slow down our inner cleansing process. With the first fallen leaf, our overall mood changes as we become exhausted with the rains and fogs all around us. Not too long ago we were enjoying the summer season, only now to be in a cooler environment with a dampened mood, a possible developing cold, and growing fatigue.

To avoid the seasonal side effects and keep a clear head, you should undergo a course of clay therapy at the end of September to help strengthen your organism and prepare you for the long winter season.

Internal application

If it is unpleasant for you to drink clay milk, then substitute it with capsules. You can consume clay capsules at any time of day. Six capsules is equivalent to about one teaspoon of clay.

Whether you choose powder, liquid, or capsules, you will still receive full benefits of clay.

For a poorly functioning digestive system, drink a clay solution in the morning on an empty stomach. Drink the solution without stirring up the settled clay powder, which will form at the bottom of the glass overnight.

For a well-functioning digestive system, drink a glass of clay milk every morning. Make sure to stir the settled clay powder before drinking.

Any course of clay treatment should begin with the start of a new lunar month and should be completed over a 21 day period. If necessary, however, it can be extended for up to three months. After three weeks, take a break for one week—completing one lunar month of a 28 day cycle. Repeat course, if necessary.

Preparing clay milk

What you will need:

- A glass

- Wooden spoon

- Mineral water

- High quality green clay powder

Instructions:

- Fill three quarters of the glass with mineral water, preferably in the evening.

- Add a full teaspoon of green clay powder.

- Stir well and leave overnight.

Precautions

Consuming clay is not recommended for people who have serious constipation or hypertension. It is also not recommended for children who are under the age of three (unless prescribed by a doctor).

Constipation:

Exercise caution if you have a history of extended periods of constipation. At the beginning of clay treatments constipation may worsen. However, gradually you should feel that your internal system will restore to a healthy state. Nevertheless, you should keep a close watch to make sure that constipation does not return and that you are regularly getting rid of all bodily waste.

Hypertension:

Likewise, exercise caution if you have a history of hypertension (*high blood pressure*). Clay supplies cells with plenty of elements, which actively help the affected vessels. During first treatments, though, clay can cause an increase in arterial blood pressure. Therefore, during the initial treatments, it is necessary to be cautious and periodically take blood pressure measurements.

External application

What is necessary to prepare a compress?

Tools

- A deep ceramic or glass dish
- Wooden spoon

- Mineral, spring or rain water

- A thin piece of fabric

- Paper napkins

- Gauze

- A roll of cellophane

Ingredients

- Sea salt (gray)

- Medicinal herbs crushed into a powder

- Infusions made from roots, flowers or leaves of medicinal herbs

- Essential oils

- Apple vinegar

- Clay

Preparing dough-like clay

- Pour some green clay granules or powder into a tray.

- Pour spring or mineral water over the clay; water level should be an inch above the clay.

- Cover with a thin fabric or napkin and leave for at least an hour.

- You can place the container in the sun since solar energy actually activates clay.

- When clay has absorbed all the water, carefully stir it with a wooden spoon to make sure there are not any dry lumps.

- Continue to stir until you have a homogeneous (*uniform*), consistency.

When properly prepared, the clay should remind you of a gentle mound of dough right before it is placed in the oven. If it has turned out too watery, then add some clay powder little by little while constantly stirring. On the other hand, if the consistency is too dense, then add mineral water. Or simpler yet, you can add water half an inch above the clay level and wait until the clay absorbs it all on its own.

How to make a compress

When clay is prepared correctly, it should be quite dense. Cover a napkin or a piece of gauze with at least a quarter of an inch layer of clay and place it on the affected area of the body. This type of compress allows you to save time.

Remove it after an hour and wipe the skin with either a wet towel or cotton ball to clean any traces of clay. It is all quite that simple. Afterwards, throw away the used clay and place the towel in the laundry.

How long to apply a compress

To reach a full medical effect, you should hold a compress in place for 2 hours. Sometimes it is recommended to leave the compress overnight; however, the ions' bioactivity typically does not last that long.

After about two hours, the ionic exchange comes to a halt and clay loses all of its activity. Also, the water evaporates during that time and clay dries up. Therefore, there is no real medical benefit to leave a compress overnight. In fact, due to its bulkiness, oftentimes a compress prevents its user from getting sleep, and proper rest is a key component to any recovery.

It is not recommended to apply a cold compress on the stomach area right after a meal because it interferes with the digestion process. As a rule of thumb, apply all compresses between meals.

How to warm up clay

The first way is to prepare dough-like clay with very hot water. Pour clay powder into a ceramic bowl and then cover it with hot water. You will hear a crackling sound as clay absorbs the water. Stir slowly until clay becomes saturated. When the clay is ready, apply it in thick layers. Clay maintains the heat of the water for quite some time.

Another way to warm clay is to lay a thick layer of ready dough-like clay on a thin napkin and then place it on a hot-water bottle. (Microwaves and ovens are poor heating options for clay.)

Initial reactions

Everyone reacts differently when first beginning to use clay. Initial reactions may occur right after the first compress is removed or even after a few days. In either case, it is helpful to be aware of all possible outcomes.

People who are new to clay therapy usually fear that their symptoms and diseases might get worse. This is especially the case with deep wounds because they may expand and become even deeper during the first stages of treatment. However, most find that soon after, the skin around the wound turns pink and begins to tighten. A few weeks further into treatment, the wound develops whitish skin signifying the beginning of a healing process.

Clay absorbs and destroys toxins while promoting a natural regeneration of skin cells and allowing wounds to tighten. Do not stop applying compresses at the first signs of healing, which may frighten you as they look like things are getting worse. Stick with it; you are on your way to recovery! Remember, clay cleanses tissues without causing any damage to a person's health.

When placing a compress to alleviate pain, the same initial reactions may occur. Pain may increase at first, as the compress reduces inflammation, but the pain should gradually subside towards the end of the session.

The healing principles are very close to thalassotherapy (*medical use of seawater as a form of therapy*). Elements in clay activate the regeneration process of damaged skin cells reducing or completely eliminating pain that stems from inflammation or trauma.

Travel with clay

Clay promotes fast healing for small cuts and wounds. Even with a bee sting, clay is able to instantly ease the pain along with the burning sensation. Therefore, it is a great idea to take a small amount of clay powder with you when you travel so that you always have it available.

The do not's of clay

- Do not use a gas oven or a microwave to heat up clay.

- Do not use any metals when working with clay or preparing clay milk, masks, or compresses because a metal can oxidize during prolonged contact.

- Do not consume clay simultaneously with medication. Clay should be taken at least 2 hours before any medication.

- Do not use tap water because it contains a lot of chlorine as well as nitrates.

- Do not add essential oils or medical products with unknown side effects.

- Do not stop. Once you begin treatment, continue without any breaks.

- Do not add paraffin oil (liquid paraffin or mineral oil) during external applications.

- Do not use plastic tools or utensils.

- Do not allow clay to dry when using it externally. Water is responsible for moving the elements into the organism.

- Do not apply a compress to skin that has been covered with cream that is anti-inflammatory or intended to warm the skin. These creams penetrate deep into the skin and, when a compress is added on top, may cause unpleasant sensations or even light burns.

- Although contrary to some opinion, do not apply clay directly to burns. Burnt skin may bubble up if clay is applied directly on it. But if you place a piece of gauze between clay and skin, it should be safe, and the therapeutic effect will not be lost. In addition, upon using gauze as a buffer, the top layer of skin cells will not be torn off when you are removing clay, which can dry up and harden around the burn before it is time to remove it. Also, you will not have to clean the wound from clay afterwards.

4

Specific Green Clay Treatments

"The reproduction of mankind is a great marvel and mystery. Had God consulted me in the matter, I should have advised him to continue the generation of the species by fashioning them out of clay." **- Martin Luther 1483-1546**

Thousands of people benefit from clay all over Russia and all over the world. The following methods have recently been used in spas and clinics throughout Russia to produce great results. Understand, however, that these results are not guaranteed for everyone, and clay treatments are not meant to substitute a consultation with your physician.

Acne

Acne is a common skin condition, characterized by areas of red scaly skin, blackheads, whiteheads, pinheads, pimples, and possibly scarring. Although it is possible to have acne at an older age as well as during hormonal imbalance, acne is most common among adolescents who especially suffer from psychological pain and misery associated with this aesthetic catastrophe.

To combat this condition, combine internal application with external.

Internal application

In addition to a physician's prescriptions, you should prepare clay milk every evening:

- Add powder clay to a glass of mineral water.

- Leave over night.

- Stir and drink in the morning.

Course of treatment can last up to three months. Furthermore, you should watch what you eat. Limit your intake of sweets, meats, and flour.

External application

Prepare a clay mask:

- Fill a cup with some green clay powder.

- Add a little bit of herbal tea made from chamomile to create a thin paste equivalent to the viscosity (*thickness*) of sour cream.

Before applying a clay mask, prepare a small steam bath for your face:

- Pour one to two quarts of water into a pot.

- Add a handful of thyme to boiling water.

- Remove the pot from the stove and put it on a sturdy surface.

- Throw a towel over your head and keep your face over the steam at a comfortable distance so as to not burn your skin.

- Keep your face over the steam for a few minutes and then pad dry.

Note: The steam is able to open up your pores and allow you to clean your skin thoroughly and on a deeper level that usual. Furthermore, thyme, a strong disinfectant, sanitizes the skin and prepares it for the mask.

Finishing up

- Remove any blackheads (*a type of acne that is a yellow or blackish bump or plug on the skin*).

- Cover your face with clay, which should have a sour cream-like consistency.

- Leave it on for 20 minutes. This should not be enough time for it to dry if the layer is thick enough. However, if you notice that it is drying, then wet a piece of gauze in the warm thyme mixture and place it on top of the mask to keep it from drying.

- After removing the mask, do not forget to use moisturizing lotion on your face.

Treatments should be conducted over a 3-5 week period. If you are showing signs of recovery, then you can lessen your sessions by half.

Aerophagia

Aerophagia results from swallowing too much air, usually while eating food. This can lead to bloating, which is sometimes painful, but more often just leads to an awkward outward appearance and discomfort.

Luckily, clay is the natural superabsorbent that you need. It is able to absorb the air swallowed involuntarily in the same way it absorbs liquid, consequently removing irritation and discomfort.

Drink a glass of clay milk daily before lunch. Course of treatment is 3 weeks. If necessary, course of treatment can be repeated.

You should actively avoid extra ingestion of air by eating slower. Also, eat fewer foods that cause gases such as dairy products.

Anemia

Anemia, a less than normal amount of blood in the body, is the most common blood disorder. When you have anemia it is common to feel fatigued, dizzy, and nauseous.

For treatment, you can either drink a glass of clay milk daily before lunch or consume capsules. Make sure to check that the clay has been sundried and that the capsules are made from natural materials if you choose to use them.

Course of treatment is 3 weeks. If you want to repeat a course, wait a week before doing so. Continue the treatment until you see considerable improvement in your condition. For a full medical effect, 3 courses of 3 weeks each are recommended.

> **Tip:** *If fatigue is accompanied by high blood pressure, try to proactively work to reduce the pressure. It is also not recommended to use clay simultaneously with other medicine — use it before or after medication.*

Angina

Angina results in heart problems and pain caused by deterioration in blood circulation and lack of oxygen in the heart (*ischemia*). The main symptom is chest pressure, a sensation that usually increases during physical activities. Furthermore, angina can cause heavy complications. Besides employing clay, you should also consult with your physician.

Internal application

To support the weakened organism, conduct a 3 week course of clay milk treatments alongside any recommendations from your therapist or physician.

External application

In addition to instructions from your physician, you can apply clay compresses:

- Clay should be made to a very thick consistency.

- First heat it and then apply to the throat. Clay may be placed on a thin piece fabric and warmed up.

- Apply 2-3 times a day.

- Keep it on for an hour.

- Change every 2 hours.

- When showing signs of improvement, you may increase the time period between sessions, ultimately, ending up with just 1-2 compresses per day.

- Course of treatment is intended for a week.

A variation of a warm compress from clay and raw cabbage leaves:

- First, it is necessary to properly prepare cabbage leaves; squeeze full leaves in your hands to make the leaves soft while causing them to let out a little bit of juice.

- Put clay on an unfolded cabbage leaf and apply it directly on the throat.

In addition to compresses, you can also do a rinse treatment:

- Pour a quart of water into a pot.

- Add alder and blackberry leaves—a handful of each.

- Boil contents for 5 minutes and allow to cool to a comfortable rinsing temperature.

- Rinse your mouth with the warm mixture up to 10 times a day.

Infusions

Cleansing the organism is recommended in any case. Make an infusion from artichoke, fumaria, and birch leaves along with cinnamon:

- Add a pinch of each to a cup.

- Add boiling water and let it brew for up to 10 minutes.

- Drink 2-3 cups a day for a month.

Fruit juice

Drink organic juices high in vitamin C, i.e. black currant and grapefruit juice.

Aphthous Ulcer (*canker sore*)

These little ulcers form around the oral cavity. And even the smallest canker sores inside the mouth can cause burning and complicate swallowing. The majority of these occur because of a malfunctioning organ within our bodies—liver, gall bladder, etc.

Internal application

Clay milk accelerates healing while cleansing our bodies of excess toxins:

- Make clay milk by adding clay powder to a glass of water and leaving it overnight.

- Drink it in the morning on an empty stomach.

- If you do not experience constipation, then drink it after stirring up the settled particles. Otherwise, just drink it without stirring.

Rinsing

Rinsing refreshes the oral cavity and accelerates healing:

- Use only boiled water.

- Add 2-3 tablespoons of clay powder to a glass of water, stir well, and rinse.

While preparing a mixture for rinsing, you can use an infusion instead of water:

- Use calendula flower—one third of an ounce per two cups of water (16oz).

- Let the infusion cool and then add 1 tablespoon of clay powder.

- Rinse 2-3 times a day for 10 days.

- Repeat the procedure every time a canker sore develops.

Flatulence (*excessive gas*)

Flatulence is a result of the inability of the digestive tract to do its job. If you are suffering from a collection of gases that cause an uncomfortable feeling in the stomach area, use clay, one of the best treatments, to absorb the gas and relieve the discomfort. Clay also improves the digestive process without interrupting the enzymes that break down food to make it available for red blood cells to absorb.

It is easy to combat excessive gas, along with the pain and uneasiness that comes with it, by following a few simple steps:

- Add a tablespoon of clay powder to noncarbonated mineral water.

- Stir and leave overnight.

- Drink in the morning on an empty stomach without stirring up the settled particles.

- After a week you can start to stir the solution before drinking it.

Tip: *If you do not like the taste, then you can take three gelatin capsules in the morning and three at noon. Duration of treatment is the same.*

You can also add an infusion to your regimen. Drink 1-2 cups of water made with anise seeds—one tablespoon per cup (8oz).

Poor Blood Circulation

Whether you apply it internally or externally, clay is an effective treatment for any age group with this problem.

Internal application

A build up of toxins and an accumulation of waste are the usual causes of blood circulation problems. Clay milk contains elements that are responsible for removing toxic substances from the organism. Drink clay milk in the morning on an empty stomach without stirring up the settled particles. Course of treatment is 3 weeks. If necessary, you can prolong the standard course of treatment by another 3 weeks or repeat it later in the year.

External application

Make a bath:

- Fill a bathtub with water temperature of about 100 °F.

- Meanwhile, prepare an infusion: Boil 2 quarts of water in a pot; add a pinch of horse chestnut bark and 2 handfuls of red grape leaves; boil for a full 10 minutes and then let it sit for just as long.

- Pour out the contents into the hot bath.

- Add a handful of clay powder—about 6-8 ounces.

- Take 10 minute baths 2-3 times a week.

Tip: *When you prepare the mixture, you may also use other herbs that stimulate blood circulation. It is recommended for you to take these baths for a few consecutive months.*

Colitis

Colitis has numerous causes, but either way it leads to problems with the gut flora (*microorganisms that live in human digestive tracts*) in the large intestine, colon, anus, etc. A fungal infection is often the first sign of an imbalance of microorganisms and leads to further complications.

Internal application

Clay captures, retains and expels microbes within an organism while restoring the micro flora (*good microorganisms*) in the intestines and strengthening the immune system. A course of treatment with green clay is recommended in all cases of colitis. Drink clay milk every morning before eating. At first you should conduct a course of treatment for 3 weeks.

Note: Be cautious when using clay milk to heal stomach problems. Go back and review the necessary steps to avoid complications.

Tip: *If you have been suffering from colitis for many years, then you should extend your course of treatment for up to 3 months. Do not hesitate to prolong the treatment as it should yield wonderful results in the end. Combine internal and external applications of clay with herbal medicine and other treatments.*

External application

To reduce inflammation, prepare a compress and apply it on the painful area. Apply 1-3 times a day for a month.

Constipation

During constipation it is very important to cleanse the intestines, thus, activating the liver and gall bladder.

To start your treatment, mix a tablespoon of clay powder into a glass of water, stir well and leave overnight to be consumed the following morning.

> **Tip:** *Cleanse your intestines by drinking 2-3 glasses of radish juice per day for 10 days. You can also make infusions. To prepare a mixture, add a teaspoon of each plant — milk thistle, althaea roots, thoroughly dried frangula bark (frangula alnus) — to a glass of mineral water. Boil 5-10 minutes. Leave to cool for 5 minutes. Use a strainer to filter out the bigger particles. Drink 2-3 cups a day.*

To restore healthy digestion and proper absorbency within the intestines, take a tablespoon of flower pollen for one and a half months. Stick to this regimen for at least a few weeks, especially if you have been suffering from constipation for a long time. Sometimes it takes as long as 2-3 months to restore the digestive tract to a well working condition.

Skin diseases

Today, there are a large number of common skin diseases including eczema, herpes, psoriasis, and dyshidrosis (*a skin condition that is characterized by small blisters on hands or feet*) among many others. Clay works well in combination with other treatments to generate great results.

Internal application

Drink clay milk, and make sure to monitor your bowel movements. If you notice developing constipation, make sure to only drink the water without stirring up the settled particles at the bottom of the glass.

After a few days of treatment, your condition may actually worsen at first while clay detaches and retains, and then expels toxins and pathogenic (*disease causing*) microorganisms which interfere with skin's functions. This is a natural effect because when clay gets to work, it penetrates deeply into the infected area. Regular course of treatment is 3 weeks.

External application

Whether the skin is dry or oozing, compresses may be directly applied with a thick layer of clay on the affected area.

Afterwards, take a bath:

- Fill your bathtub. The water should not be too hot.

- Add 1 quart of an infusion made with burdock leaves.

- Add about a half of a pound of large sea salt.

- Take a bath for 20 minutes 2-3 times a week.

Tips: *The dissolved elements in the water penetrate into the skin for a deep cleansing. If you have eczema, after the first bath, it is normal to develop some sensitivity or even pain.*

Precautions

- During a sudden inflammation or an incredible itch in the case of eczema, you should immediately supplement your medical treatment with green clay compresses.

- If the bath is prepared for a child, do not add salt.

- If you have dyshidrosis, especially on the soles of your feet, the bubble formations on your skin may grow in size and even burst. During these circumstances you should apply a thick compress, and change it often throughout the day.

- Skin diseases usually require a lengthy treatment, which becomes tedious and frustrating, but the end result is well worth it in the end. Ultimately, you only need to sacrifice a month of your time for the entire course of treatment to experience incredible results.

Diarrhea

There are numerous causes for diarrhea, some of which can have terrible consequences. Consult with your family doctor since further analysis can reveal the true characteristics of your problem.

Whether you are about to go on vacation or you have just come back from a country where diarrhea is common, you should immediately buy some illite green clay. You will not regret that you did. Even the slightest intestinal problems will become a thing of the past when you use it. Clay will save you from those unpleasant moments that may ruin your trip as you will end up reading the encryptions on the bathroom stalls rather than the map if you forgo this simple treatment.

During the first signs of symptoms, do not delay and begin treatment immediately and continue it for several days. If you have further complications, then you may continue treatment for up to 21 days. In case of a relapse—when there are no serious complications in the intestines—you may extend treatment with clay milk anywhere from two months to a half a year.

Cleansing the organism

If you notice that you are developing poor blood circulation, problems digesting food, an increase in cellulite and liver troubles, then it is a good time to start thinking about cleansing your organism. In these instances clay is a simple and an effective way to restore your health. While supplying the organism with the necessary elements, clay is also able to rid the body of toxic substances, which initially caused the harm.

Drink a glass of clay milk in the morning on an empty stomach. Just after the first week your organism functions should improve. You will notice the improvement through an increase in energy. It means that the organism managed to cope with an overabundance of toxic substances and is on its way to restoring its equilibrium.

Course of treatment is at least three months. If necessary, it can be prolonged.

Duodenitis *(duodenum inflammation)*

If you do not suffer from constipation in the slightest bit, then you can stir well before drinking a glass of clay milk in the mornings. Course of treatment is at least 3 weeks. If necessary, you may take a week break and repeat the entire course or until full recovery.

If you experience constipation at any time, then you should stop stirring the settled particles and just drink the solution as it is. Once your digestive system returns to its normal process, you can start stirring again.

Indigestion

Indigestion happens when the stomach is unable to properly process food. Symptoms include upper stomach pain and varying degrees of heartburn.

If you wish to improve or restore your digestive system, then you will first need to start eating a balanced diet which should include easily digestible products. Furthermore, you should conduct a course of clay treatment. Clay gently stimulates and regulates your digestion system helping it to break down food.

Keep in mind that the effect of clay is not felt until after a few weeks of treatment. But when it is, you should notice a tremendous improvement in your digestion as well as reduced bloating and pain while your fatigue will be replaced with vibrant energy.

Depending on your body's response and your lifestyle choices, the course of treatment can last as long as a year.

> **Tips**: *Treating indigestion demands a well-hydrated organism. Drink as much water as possible.*

Fatigue

Fatigue can creep up in many different situations: at the end of a pregnancy, the beginning of winter, or after a long battle with an illness. Rich with minerals, clay strengthens an organism and restores vitality. Take it daily to help regain life and vigor. Do not, however, attempt to overcome fatigue all at once, but instead try to structure a step-by-step course of treatment.

Prepare clay milk and leave it overnight. If you do not suffer from constipation, then stir settled particles in the morning before drinking clay milk on an empty stomach. Course of treatment is 3 weeks, and can be repeated several times a year.

> **Tips:** *Be sure to seek the right effect — a smooth flow of energy — instead of just a state of excitement, which can once again leave you feeling tired and weary afterwards.*

Along with clay milk, also drink fresh organic fruit juices rich with vitamin C.

Severe, chronic, extreme fatigue

If you are suffering from extreme fatigue to the point where you are not able to sleep, experience high blood pressure, a ringing in your ears, or smooth muscle spasms, then clay has certain advantages as a choice of treatment because it has numerous elements, which can help to stabilize the functions of your organism.

Prepare a glass of clay milk in the evening by adding a teaspoon of clay powder to a glass of mineral water. Drink it in the mornings on an empty stomach without stirring. Continue treatment for a minimum of 3 weeks.

Hepatitis

Hepatitis is an inflammation of the liver. There are various forms of hepatitis and various causes. When you experience a slight pain in the area of the liver or even more serious symptoms of this disease, there are several approaches to treatment.

Internal application

Green clay is one of the best supplements to modern medicinal treatments of hepatitis. Clay strengthens the defense systems of an organism, while providing a deep and intense cleansing, especially during viral hepatitis.
Treatments can be lengthy—half a year and sometimes even more. Also, it is necessary for you to keep a close track of your bowel movements to avoid complications.

External application

Clay penetrates into the skin, removes toxins and gradually reduces inflammation. It is necessary for you to do compresses long before taking your medication (if you have a prescription for one).

Prepare a compress:

- Prepare a thick mixture of clay that resembles the density of dough.

- Wrap it in a piece of gauze.

- Apply it to the area of the liver.

- You may keep it there for up to an hour.

- To achieve a full medical effect, you need to conduct compresses daily for at least 3 months.

Diaphragmatic hernia

Diaphragmatic hernia is a hole in the diaphragm that allows the abdominal contents to escape into the chest cavity. It often happens to people who are under constant stress. Hernias usually do not heal on their own, and most often require surgery. But it is possible to lessen the discomfort with clay.

It should not take long for you to feel its effect. During the beginning stages, you will have a feeling of increased discomfort, however, the pain and belching will gradually begin to fade and eventually disappear.

Drink a glass of clay milk every morning on an empty stomach. Course of treatment is at least 3 months.

Restoring the right balance of mineral salts

Restoring the right balance of minerals salts is absolutely necessary when facing any type of bone disease and during pain from inflammation. The process of ionic exchange helps clay to saturate bones with minerals.

A simple course of treatment with clay can allow you to restore the right balance of calcium and magnesium, helping to eliminate pain, especially if it stems from the joints.

If you prepare a glass of clay milk in the morning, then it will be ready for you to drink before lunch time. For the first few sessions just drink the water without stirring the settled particles.

Continue the course of treatment for 3 weeks. Take a break for a week and then repeat. You may also combine clay milk with compresses.

This course of treatment can be very useful for future mothers. During pregnancy, women oftentimes experience a deficiency in minerals, which may lead to some ugly consequences: loss of hair, brittle nails, deteriorating teeth, growing stress and fatigue.

A multi-week treatment with clay may resolve the root of these kinds of problems. Young mothers, who aim to avoid mineral deficiency, are taking part in this treatment with tremendous results.

Stress

During stress and physical fatigue, follow the regular course of treatment:

- Mix a teaspoon of green clay—hopefully a type with high-cleansing abilities is available to you—into a glass of water.

- Leave overnight.

- If you do not suffer from constipation, stir in the morning and drink.

- Continue for 3 weeks.

- If necessary to repeat, do so after a one week break.

This course of treatment works best during spring and fall.

Ulcers

There are a number of different types of ulcers: stomach ulcers; venous ulcers *(during varicose veins)*; ulcers caused by burns; not healing ulcers, etc.

Internal application

If you are suffering from a stomach ulcer, then results are usually better if you start treatment sooner rather than later. Drink a glass of clay milk in the mornings on an empty stomach and the ulcer should gradually begin to heal.

Note: At first, you may feel a burning sensation which will gradually fade away and should completely disappear after a month of treatment.

External application

The reasons of the occurrence of ulcers include genetic predisposition, not healing wounds, or the illnesses caused by various functional infringements on the work of an organ.

Bedsores

Bedsores are very difficult to treat and are extremely painful. Most often they happen to the elderly who lie in bed in one place for a long period of time without any movement. These ulcers also oftentimes lead to scabs.

Besides internal treatment with clay, it is necessary to take preventative measures with inch-thick compresses under the affected area of the back. During first signs of scabs, prepare a thick layer of a compress and change it regularly during the day; although, the compress can actually be left on for 2-3 days, provided that it remains soft and moist.

Continue treatment until all scabs are dissolved. This process is usually anywhere from two weeks up to one and a half months. To prevent a formation of new scabs, continue to place fresh compresses underneath the back of the patient.

Simple ulcers

Apply a compress on the affected area when faced with more simple ulcers, such as the ones caused by burns.

Apply clay directly on the skin or place some gauze in between. The latter choice allows you to forgo washing the wound which can be painful in certain circumstances.

Compresses should cover the entire affected area of the skin and should be applied for at least an hour. Do not allow the skin to dry. You can further help to keep the skin moist by applying chamomile oil.

Abscess

Abscess, a collection of pus that collects in any part of the body, is created by the body's defense system during an infection that may result from a cut, a small wound, or a variety of tooth problems.

An abscess is usually very painful and requires immediate attention:

- Prepare dough-like clay.

- Add a drop of thyme and lavender essential oils per 3.5 oz.

- Carefully mix and apply a thick layer of clay directly on the abscess. Note: To apply a compress to more difficult places like fingers and toes, create dough-like clay in a tall cup and then submerge your toe or finger in the mix.

- It is necessary to apply 5-6 times a day. Sometimes, towards the end of the day, the wound will break open causing the pus to come out. This can be quite painful. But even if the pain is very strong, you should not remove the compress.

- Continue to do applications for 2-3 days until the abscess disappears.

Tips: *To relieve pain, prepare a tray with an infusion of boiled boxwood leaves and add a handful of grey sea salt. After each compress, soak (or rinse) the abscess 2-3 times.*

Arthritis

Arthritis is an inflammation of the joints, accompanied by sharp pain. Carry out an auxiliary course of healing with clay compresses:

- Boil a quart of water.

- Add a handful of thyme and a handful of rosemary.

- Use this infusion to prepare the clay.

- Wrap the prepared clay in a thin napkin or a piece of gauze and apply it gently on the point of pain.

- Leave it on for two hours.

- You can repeat 3-5 times a day.

Several weeks will pass before pain should begin to subside. Patiently continue the treatment. After some time you should feel that you have a lot more mobility and a lot less pain. Meanwhile, you should also apply clay internally.

Osteoarthritis

It is typical to find osteoarthritis in the joints of the elbows, knees, and shoulders, as well as in the backbone—in particular, cervical vertebrae. Upon affecting the joints in the legs, osteoarthritis can cause serious problems with everyday movement. Besides stiffness and pain, this disease can be accompanied by dizziness and a ringing in the ears.

It is necessary to consult with a doctor. Afterwards, you can supplement the prescribed treatment with clay compresses:

- Clay can be applied directly or through a thin napkin or fabric.

- Apply a thick layer of clay on the painful area.

- Make daily applications and keep them on for 2 hours. If the situation suddenly worsens, you can increase the number of daily applications to 3.

- The duration of treatment depends on the illness. Be prepared for at least 3 months of intense treatment.

During osteoarthritis, especially during a sudden aggravation, your organism really needs the elements which are contained in clay. Combine external applications with internal applications and make sure to monitor your bowel movements.

Burns

There are different degrees of burns. First degree burns can be healed with clay. Second, third and fourth degree burns require medical treatment and sterile conditions.

First degree burns may happen in a variety of ways: little skin bubbles filled with water forming from wearing tight shoes; boiling water or acid spilled on skin; and sunburn.

When burned, it is important to act quickly. Always have some clay powder nearby. The skin will usually turn red following a light burn, which can be immediately treated with a compress:

- First rinse the wound with a slow stream of warm water, which, preferably, should be body temperature. Carefully get the wound wet, and do not wipe it dry.

- Put a piece of gauze on the burn and a thick layer of clay on top for 10 minutes.

- Replace it and keep it on for another 10 minutes.

- It is important to do 5 applications per day. Clay should instantly counteract pain and the burning sensation.

Cellulite

Without getting into too many detailed descriptions, many people agree that cellulite looks bad. Most people refer to it as orange peel skin or cottage cheese skin, to say the least. When you can see those bumps, it simply means that your body is doing a poor job of cleaning out the toxins in your blood. Your doctor should easily spot poor blood circulation and prescribe a treatment. You can supplement that treatment with a daily glass of clay milk in the mornings.

You can also take 2-3 clay baths a weeks:

- Fill a bath tub with 100 °F water.

- On the side, boil water with leaves for 10 minutes. Include a handful of each: grape, rosemary, and cypress leaves. Pour out the contents into the bath.

- Add 2-4 lbs of clay powder and enjoy.

Note: Make sure to stir the clay well so as not to clog up the drain pipe.

Bruises and traumas

No matter how the trauma occurred—falling from a bicycle, hitting your finger with a hammer, bruising or swollen bump due to a hit or punch—a clay compress can be an effective treatment. Apply it directly on the skin or through some gauze and hold it in place for an hour.

To treat a bruise, it is enough to do 3-6 applications a day for 2 days. If you have a large hematoma (*localized collection of blood outside the blood vessels that can be seen by skin discoloration as it turns blue, black, and yellow*), you should continue applications for at least 6 days in a row. You will notice hematoma change colors as it gradually dissolves.

Note: Make sure to wait until stitches are removed to apply compresses following postoperative trauma.

Pain of various sources

To remove pain of whatever origin—postoperative or rheumatic—the approach is the same, although the duration of treatment may vary.

Prepare clay and apply it either directly to the skin or through gauze:

- During insignificant pain—a light hit, a fall, or a slight trauma—a course of treatment lasts 1-2 weeks.

- During strong traumatic or rheumatic pain, the course of treatment is prolonged up to half a year. During treatment, the pain should gradually subside and/or occur less frequently.

- In some medical institutions, methods of clay treatment have been accepted for a long time. When experiencing pain after an operation, whether it is in the area of the mouth, a meniscus or the abdominal cavity, wait until the doctor clears you to use clay compresses, which may promote the dissolving of post-operative hematomas.

Note: Do not apply compresses over stitches or following plastic surgery.

Muscle pains and aches

You can either make a bath or apply a compress:

- Pour one quart of boiling water over 4 ounces of Fraxinus (ash) leaves and let it cool.

- Add the solution to clay powder until you get a dough-like consistency.

- Apply an inch thick layer directly to the affected area and leave it on for an hour.

- Apply 2-3 times a day for 1-2 weeks.

Calluses

To treat a callus, apply compresses daily:

- Peel a lemon.

- Cut the peel into small pieces—a quarter to a half of an inch.

- Soak the lemon peels in apple vinegar for two days.

- After preparing the lemon peels with this method, apply them to the callus to soften the skin.

- Top it off with a ball of prepared clay, which should be the size of a grape.

- Apply for 15 minutes 2-3 times a day.

- Each time take off the soft top layer of skin.

- Continue the process until the callus disappears.

Warts

Plantar warts are often removed through surgery. Yet, depending on the affected area and a weakness of the immune system, they oftentimes return after a few months. Their roots are so deep that the surgeon is usually forced to penetrate far into the affected area to try to eliminate the wart in its entirety.

Clay compresses should free you from the inconvenience of an operation along with all the worries and the costs. Furthermore, you will not have to trade one ugly site for another— a wart for a scar. It will seem as though the wart drowned in clay as it cleans, disinfects and regenerates the epidermis (*top layer*) of the skin. And best of all, if done correctly, you should not have to deal with it ever again.

Planter wart treatments, although more difficult and lengthy, can also be accomplished with a compress:

- Prepare dough-like clay and apply a thick layer on the wart.

- Leave it on for half an hour to an hour.

- Make daily applications. Each time take off the softened top layer of the skin along with the exposed wart roots.

- Continue treatment for 1-3 weeks.

- Stop the treatment when you no longer see black dots (wart roots) on the skin.

Daily hand skincare is essential. Unfortunately, warts can develop on your fingers and hands. If you are lucky enough to have a fig tree growing in your yard, then you have the most simple and natural source at your disposal to treat these warts. Use the ripening fruits alongside green clay compresses for an accelerated healing process.

To treat all other warts, regularly swab them with fig juice—plenty of it comes out from a small incision in a fresh fig.

After a few procedures you will feel light prickling and burning. After a few weeks, however, of regular applications of clay and fresh fig juice, the wart should disappear.

Frostbite

Frostbite most often strikes fingertips, toes, chin and nose.

Prepare a tray for treatment:

- Mix a pound of clay powder with a burdock leaf infusion.

- Submerge the affected area into the tray of clay.

- Keep it there for 20 minutes.

- Afterwards, rinse with warm water, dry and apply extremely oily cream.

- Make 1-2 trays a day for 2 weeks.

Tips: *In addition to clay compresses, apply cabbage leaves. Put crushed cabbage leaves on the affected area for an hour. Do 2 applications per day for 2 weeks in order to help renew your skin and regain smoothness.*

Erythema in the area of the buttocks

Erythema is a reddening and irritation of the skin caused by hyperemia (*congestion of blood*) in the capillaries. In this case, green clay is used in its dry powder form to help remove the initial burning pain. If the condition has progressed to a point where clay is unable to remove the pain, then you can still use clay to help restrict further inflammation and restore the pH level of the top layer of the skin (*the epidermis*) while accelerating the recovery process.

For infants who are suffering from a fever due to teething, clay is helpful in getting rid of pain and allowing the infant to quickly fall asleep. During significant reddening you can use a slightly different approach:

- Boil water with boxwood leaves—1 ounce of leaves per 4 ounces of water.

- Let it cool.

- Soak a cotton ball in the prepared solution and wipe the infant's buttocks in the morning and evening.

- You can also apply a compress made from the same mixture by adding it to clay powder. Within a few hours the inflammation should go away.

Sprains

Sprains usually happen in an area of ankles, wrists, and shoulders. In any case, it is necessary to apply very dense clay and cover the entire area of pain. Place a half-an-inch thick layer of clay on the skin with gauze in between. Often, the injured area is not comfortable for maintaining a compress, so you should tie it down with a bandage. Do it daily for 1-2 hours for at least a month.

In the beginning, there is a possibility that the pain will intensify, but do not worry as it should soon lessen or disappear altogether.

Dry, cracking skin on hands

Small cracks in the skin may appear as a result of a vitamin deficiency or cold temperature. Help yourself to a compress:

- Use 4-7 ounces of clay powder and a glass of mineral water to prepare a dough-like clay mixture. Make it thinner and less dense than usual.

- Add lemon juice and olive oil—a tablespoon of each.

- Either apply the compress directly on the affected area or place a piece of gauze in between.

- Applications can be made 2-3 times a day for 15 minutes. Do not allow the clay to dry.

- Wash off your hands and apply a small amount of olive oil.

- Continue the treatment for 1-2 weeks.

Cracking skin on the nipple

If little cracks form on your nipples while breastfeeding, make a compress:

- Boil 2 ounces of comfrey roots in a quart of water.

- Allow to cool down.

- Create a mix of very dense dough-like clay. To attain a dense mixture, pour very slowly while constantly stirring.

- Take a small piece and apply it through gauze on the nipple.

- Hold it in place for an hour.

- Make 2-3 applications per day and continue treatment for 1-2 weeks.

- Between compresses apply avocado oil.

5

Cosmetic Applications with Green Clay

"A thing of beauty is a joy forever" - **John Keats (1975-1821)**

Rich with bioactive elements, clay clears up rashes, scabs, etc., while whitening and removing blemishes from all skin types—oily, normal, dry. Clay helps restore pH levels, get rid of pimples, and regulate sebaceous glands (*microscopic glands in the skin that secrete an oily/ waxy matter, called sebum, to lubricate the skin and hair*). Furthermore, external applications of clay activate and rejuvenate nerve endings on the surface of the skin.

The elements within clay supply skin with nutrients, allowing it to restore its normal functions. Silicon, one of the main elements in clay, penetrates into the cellular membrane (*outer shell*), where it is much needed for everyday cell functions. Calcium and magnesium participate in cell regeneration. Selenium, although present in small doses, slows down the cellular aging process. Chromium takes part in supplying oxygen to cells.

Ultimately, green clay has a great value for organisms in its entirety because its chemical makeup is very similar to our own. So, with all these benefits, why not use clay to help our organisms?

Facial skincare

Although most people know that clay is great for oily, shiny skin, it is also great for other types: gentle, sensitive, dry and cracking, and that which is covered with rashes, pimples, acne, and scabs.

Clay is a great source of health for your skin. Put it on your face at any time of day. Just make sure that it does not dry; keep wet cotton balls nearby to moisten the clay mask if necessary. After 15-20 minutes remove the mask and apply a moisturizing cream.

Deep face wash for oily skin

- Get a clean cup.

- Add a teaspoon of green clay powder.

- Add a teaspoon of ground almonds.

- Add mineral water or cornflower extract and stir while pouring to reach a sour cream-like consistency.

- Apply liberally to your face with light strokes and circular movements.

- Gently massage the clay into the tip of the nose, forehead, and chin.

- Afterwards, wash away with water.

- Then apply a cleansing mask.

- Afterwards, apply moisturizing cream.

Deep face wash for normal skin

- Get a clean cup.

- Add a tablespoon of green clay powder.

- Add a teaspoon of ground apricot kernels.

- Mix in orange blossom extract until you get a sour cream-like consistency.

- Gently massage the mask into your facial skin with light strokes and circular movements.

- Afterwards, wash away with water, dry, and apply moisturizing cream.

Cleansing mask for oily skin

- Get a clean cup.

- Add 3 tablespoons of green clay powder.

- Extract juice from half a cucumber.

- While stirring, slowly pour cucumber juice to create a sour cream-like consistency.

- Apply liberally.

- On the more oily areas—forehead, nose, and chin—place thin slices of cucumber.

- Leave it on for 20 minutes.

- Wash it off with warm water, dry, and apply moisturizing cream.

Start your treatment with 2 sessions a week until you see improvement, and then you can decrease it to just one session a week. Continue to make and apply this mask from time to time throughout the year. It can play a significant role in regulating your sebaceous glands.

Cleansing mask for all types of skin

- Prepare your face by rubbing it down with makeup-removing milk.

- Get a clean cup.

- Thoroughly mix 2 tablespoons of green clay powder and 1 teaspoon of almonds ground into powder.

- Add a drop of fresh squeezed orange juice.

- Gently massage clay into your skin by making circular movements with your fingertips giving special attention to your nose and chin.

- Allow the mask to sit for 5-10 minutes.

- Remove it with cosmetic wipes.

- Wash the rest off with warm water.

- Do not forget to apply cream designed for your skin type immediately afterwards.

Whitening mask

Green clay possesses strong whitening properties that can help you to remove blemishes, sunspots or unwanted freckles. You will need several things to make a mask:

- 2 full tablespoons of illite green clay.

- A pinch of oatmeal soaked in hot milk.

- 4-5 drops of essential oils.

- Mix thoroughly and let it sit for 15 minutes.

- Before applying the mask, soak flowers of wild pansies.

- After the mask is applied, soak cotton balls in the prepared infusion and put them on the center part of the face—nose, forehead, and chin. Hold them there for several minutes.

- Keep the mask on for 10-15 minutes and then wash your face, dry it, and apply moisturizing cream.

Acne skincare mask

- Prepare an infusion of one glass of water and a pinch of burdock leaves and wild pansy flowers.

- Get a clean cup.

- Add a tablespoon of green clay powder.

- Add a tablespoon of the prepared infusion.

- Add a full teaspoon of oatmeal.

- Mix it all together and apply to the affected areas only.

- Leave it on for 20 minutes.

- Wash your face off with the remaining infusion.

- Dry your face and then use the remaining clay to cover your entire face.

- Leave it on for 15 minutes.

- Take off the mask and then apply moisturizing cream.

- Repeat this procedure 3-4 times a week.

Green clay accelerates the healing process and improves skin tone, helping to make it smooth and velvety, while also returning a healthy glow to your face. It is beneficial to combine masks with internal clay applications.

Tips: *Clay deeply penetrates into the skin; thus, cleaning the skin and removing acne. Usually acne disappears after a few days. The most important part is not to stop the treatment.*

Body skincare

Weight loss bath

Do not overlook a medicinal bath as a means to shed some weight and regain your beautiful figure, which you may have lost over the winter period or during pregnancy.

- Make a bath with 2 pounds of clay. While green clay is the best choice, you can also use red or white clay.

- On the side, boil a big pot of water with a handful of rosemary leaves and red grape leaves and half of a handful of black current leaves.

- Add the solution to the bath.

- You can also add aromatherapy of your choice to the medicinal herbs and clay. There is a wide variety to choose from; lavender essential oil, fruit incense, mint, and so on.

- Take 20 minute baths 3-4 times a week.

Submerge yourself into the bath; experience the pleasure of the sweet aroma and the healing process in action.

For self-encouragement, before and after baths, keep a diary of your waist size. This way you can measure the effectiveness of the treatment.

Relaxing bath

Life is full of stress. To help you find internal harmony and to feel good about yourself, take a relaxing bath:

- Add a handful of greed clay powder.

- Add 10 drops of essential oils—lavender, rosemary, and orange blossom extract. Essential oils play a key role in relaxation.

- Now submerge yourself in these amazing, pleasant waters.

- Enjoy for 20 minutes and then take a refreshing shower.

Stimulating bath

When you are slightly tired or hung over after a late night out, it would be nice to feel refreshed and reenergized:

- Pour a hot bath of approximately 100 °F.

- At same time, on the side, prepare an infusion by adding handfuls of thyme, rosemary, and sage to a quart of boiling water.

- Filter out the leaves and pour the infusion into the bath.

- Add green clay.

- Submerge your body and prepare to have a great day.

A bath to improve blood circulation

If you have noticed some problems with your blood circulation, then you may need to take a medicinal bath:

- Prepare a hot bath.

- Boil 2 quarts of water on the side.

- Add some horse chestnut bark, red grape leaves, and a handful of crushed seaweed.

- Dissolve 1 pound of green clay in the infusion and pour it out into the bath.

- Make sure the water temperature is not too hot so as not to get burned. This bath, however, should cause you to sweat heavily. Active substances in the bath should further stimulate the blood circulation and expel toxins in the process.

- You may take 2-3 baths a week.

Softening bath (for skin diseases)

For psoriasis, eczema, and other various types of skin irritants, you need to make a cold infusion:

- For 2-3 quarts of water add a handful of burdock leaves, a handful of calendula flowers, and two handfuls of oatmeal.

- Pour out the infusion into the bath.

- Add 2 pounds of green clay powder and a few drops of myrrh essential oil.

- The temperature should be moderate—below 100 °F.

- Take this bath for 15 minutes 2 times a week. Combine it with other treatments.

Clay mask for the body

- Prepare a mix from 2 full tablespoons of wheat germ and a handful of oatmeal.

- Prior to creating the mix, soak the oatmeal in water (1 cup) and apple vinegar (½ cup).

- Pour 2 pounds of green clay powder into a large pot.

- Add the mix and stir until you reach a homogenous consistency.

- Slowly pour heated mineral water while mixing.

- Prepare a very hot bath.

- Add 1 pound of pink clay, a few drops of lavender oil, and orange blossom extract.

- Before stepping into the bath, apply the prepared clay on the body while giving special attention to those areas that need the most therapy.

- When you feel that you are starting to become stiff as the clay dries, dip into the bath, and make sure to enjoy the next few pleasant moments that it will give to you.

You should feel great afterwards and your
skin should feel velvety and smooth.

These preparations may seem labor intensive, but do
not skip the body mask as it can give you great results.
Sometimes you just want to improve how you feel. And
clay helps to make that possible.

Mask for the chest

If you wish to tighten up your sagging, drooping breasts,
then the following recipe can help:

- Pour 1 pound of well-filtered green clay
  powder in a cup.

- Prepare a warm glass of water and add 10
  drops of garden savory essential oil, 2-3
  drops of sage essential oil, and 1-2 drops
  of lavender essential oil.

- Pour this glass out into the cup with clay
  in it. Stir until the mixture is homogenous
  with a sour cream-like consistency.

- Cover your breasts with gauze soaked in a
  cold infusion made with sage and parsley.

- Then place a thick layer of clay over the
  gauze and top it off with another layer of
  gauze soaked in the same cold infusion.

- Keep it there for 45 minutes.

- Remove it and wipe with cosmetic wipes.

- You can make 2-3 masks a week.

6

Different Colored Clay

"Beauty awakens the soul to act." **- Dante Alighieri**

"Everybody needs beauty as well as bread, places to play in and pray in, where nature may heal and give strength to body and soul." **-John Muir (1838-1914)**

Ability to oxidize is one of the most important properties of clay. The color of clay mainly depends on the oxides entering its structure. In particular, it is colored by iron oxide. Red, yellow, and brown clay contain iron oxides which define the clay's color scale. White clay, however, is an exception, largely in part because of its high aluminum content—more than 25%. It is the aluminum that gives clay a silver-white color.

However, not only colorful oxides determine the color of clay. The color is also influenced by the set of minerals within. (To explain this phenomenon in detail would take quite some time.)

Pink, white, red, and yellow clay contain elements that promote skin cell regeneration; they tone, whiten, and soften the skin while getting rid of irritants. These types of clay have a low cation exchange capacity and, furthermore, help the skin maintain a constant and healthy level of pH.

Pink clay

Pink clay is a mix of red and white koalinite clay. They give clay a gentle-pink color, pleasant for cosmetic use. Pink clay is richer in elements than white clay, yet it maintains its softness and neutrality due to white koalinite contents. And the layered structure allows it to be a good absorbent.

Pink clay is usually applied for cosmetic purposes and mainly to make masks. It is great for cosmetic care of sensitive skin. It is also great for dry and aging skin. Pink clay is only partially sundried because white clay is extracted by the ton and cannot be fully subjected to sunrays. (Only red clay is completely sundried.)

White clay

White clay, or koalinite, is the most known of the colored clays. Within its structure it posses aluminum that does not have active ions and the ions do not enter into ionic exchange. Thus, for the most part, this clay is inert and inactive—the tape structure does not promote ionic exchange either. (Also, white clay is scarce in elements compared to others.)

White clay is usually obtained from a mine and is seldom white; instead it is oftentimes silver-white. It is cleaned in gigantic containers, filtered and dried in drums designed for that purpose. But no matter where it is mined, it usually has no impurities, quickly hydrates, and has a low shrink-swell capacity.

It is most often applied with cosmetic purposes to sensitive skin and remains in high demand among women. Some of the best results can be achieved with high-quality white clay extracted in France. Put a thin layer of white clay on your face; it will quickly dry up, creating a thin white coating which smoothes the skin.

White clay is used to manufacture cosmetic products because it combines well with various components. For example, it is a key component of baby powders. The most widespread use of white clay, however, is in manufacturing ceramics and animal feed.

Red clay

Red clay is a part of many groups of clay minerals: illite, koalinite, and smectite. Iron oxide gives the clay its rusty-brown color. It has a layered structure and this structure of elements closely resembles green illite and montmorillonite. To determine quality, look for the "sundried" on the packing label.

This clay is often prepared for various masks and baths as it renders incredible softening results. It also possesses the right properties to whiten and tone. Applied only externally, red clay is usually recommended for oily, sensitive skin.

Yellow clay

For many years people have used yellow clay to take care of their face. It belongs to the same illite group and has the same elements. During oxidation—the same process as in red clay—it develops iron oxides; the cleansing properties of yellow clay, however, are stronger than red clay even though they share the same layered structure.

In comparison to other clays, yellow clay has a very high absorbency and is extremely active when in contact with the epidermis. Yellow clay is great for normal, slightly oily and sensitive skin types.

Quality color clays

Rest assured that when you use color clays for masks or medical mud baths, they do not disturb the pH balance of the skin and, therefore, hardly ever cause irritation or allergic reactions. Quality color clay is just as good as other clay. Before being sold in stores, they go through similar quality control tests and inspections to make sure that the consumer is receiving something good.

Their mineralogical structure is often homogeneous and includes ions and calcium cations (*a soft white element which is found in bones, teeth, and many other natural structures*), magnesium, silicon, and potassium. The ionic exchange is weak, however. And for the most part these clays are soft and neutral; hence, they are used for cosmetic purposes and in other industries as base components for different products.

Color clay has very similar properties as other clay and easily combines with various other masks and baths. The following is a selection of recipes for masks from red, pink, white, and yellow clay.

Facial skincare

All the described masks are quite "light" and should not cause any discomfort or damage to your skin. You can apply them 1-2 times a month. So that your mask will not dry, you can top it off with gauze soaked in clay milk made from the same clay as your mask.

A deep facial cleanse for normal skin

- Pour a tablespoon of red clay into a cup.

- Add mineral water and a teaspoon of ground germ of wheat.

- Continue to mix until you have a homogenous sour cream-like consistency.

- Apply a thick layer of clay all over your face, including around the eyes.

- Slowly massage your face in circular movements with your fingertips.

- The mask helps remove the dead cells accumulated on the top layer of your skin, and smoothes out rough patches of skin to give it extra elasticity and flexibility.

- Make this mask 1-2 times a month depending on the condition of your skin.

- After a cleansing mask, make a mask to whiten and soften your skin.

A deep facial cleanse for dry or mature skin

A green clay mask, which slightly dehydrates the skin, may pose a danger for gentle and sensitive skin types. For this type of skin, it is more suitable to use another color of clay:

- Get a clean cup.

- Add 2 full tablespoons of white clay, 1 tablespoon of lightly ground almonds and 1 tablespoon of lightly ground wheat germ.

- Mix while adding a thin stream of mineral water to reach a sour cream-like density.

- Apply evenly to your face.

- Use your fingertips to massage lightly with circular movements for several minutes.

- Remove the mask with wet cosmetic wipes and then dry your face.

- Now apply a white clay mask to soften your skin.

- Afterwards apply moisturizing cream.

Mask for acne covered skin

- Pour 3 full tablespoons of white clay powder into a cup.

- Add a teaspoon of chamomile oil.

- Add a teaspoon of wheat germ and some warm water until you reach a sour cream-like consistency.

- Apply a thick mask for 20 minutes without letting it dry. You can keep a spray bottle nearby to humidify your mask when necessary.

- Use cosmetic wipes to remove your mask.

- Do not forget to use nourishing and moisturizing cream afterwards.

- Make 1-2 masks a month.

Mask for irritable skin

If your skin is becoming more and more sensitive and/or you are experiencing sudden allergic reactions, there can be several causes including an unhealthy diet, new synthetic cosmetics, etc. To combat your reactions, use color clay and prepare a mask.
White clay is the preferred choice because it is neutral and combines well with various essential oils.

- Pour some white clay powder into a cup.

- Add two drops of lavender essential oil, and a spoonful of grape seed oil.

- Instead of water, add fresh strawberry juice.

- Apply a thick layer for 10 minutes without letting it dry.

- Remove with cosmetic wipes soaked in clean water.

- Afterwards, use moisturizing cream.

Mask for mature skin

Aging—thin, wrinkled, flabby, irritable—skin especially demands good care. Use masks that help to tone and whiten your skin and regulate its pH levels:

- Get a clean cup.

- Add 2 tablespoons of white clay powder.

- Dissolve 10 drops of chamomile essential oil and a drop of sage oil in a cup with some warm water.

- Mix with care to make sure that the mix does not end up too runny.

- Apply a thick layer to your face for 10 minutes.

- Wash off with water, dry, and apply nourishing and moisturizing cream.

Mask for dry and irritable skin

Having cleansed your face, you can now apply a mask to whiten, tone, and moisturize your skin:

- Get a clean cup.

- Add 2 full tablespoons of pink clay powder.

- Add 2 drops of sage oil and 1 drop of lavender oil.

- Mix the essential oils with warm water and afterwards mix it in with the clay.

- Stir well and apply for 15 minutes.

- In the summertime, cover your mask with moistened orange blossoms or cotton balls soaked in a cold infusion made with linden flowers.

- Remove the mask, dry your face, and apply nourishing cream.

- You can make this mask twice a month.

Mask for sensitive skin

Sensitive skin, having characteristics of dryness and redness, tends to be very irritable. Even during slightly cold weather it is quick to become quite red. Help yourself to a mask:

- Get a clean cup.

- Add 2 full tablespoons of pink clay powder.

- Add a teaspoon of chamomile oil to warm water and some drops of avocado oil.

- Then, add some mineral water and pour it all into the cup containing the clay.

- Apply the clay, which should have a sour cream-like density, on the surface of your skin and keep it there for 10 minutes.

- Top it off with gauze soaked in warm water.

- Remove the mask with the help of cosmetic wipes and apply moisturizing cream.

- You can make this mask 2 times a month preferably in the summer time.

Mask for dry and peeling skin

If you have dry, sensitive and highly irritable skin, and the skin around your eyebrows, forehead and lips is peeling, you should make a mask that softens and cleanses. See the directions for cleansing applications earlier in the chapter and then apply this softening mask to your face:

- Pour 2 tablespoons of white or pink clay powder into a cup.

- Add a tablespoon of chamomile extract, and a few drops of almond oil.

- Stir well until you form a homogenous consistency resembling sour cream.

- Put it on your face and leave it on for 15 minutes.

- Remove with cosmetic wipes soaked in warm water.

- Dry your face and do not forget to use revitalizing cream at the end.

Mask for normal skin

This mask will give your face a fresh and healthy glow:

- Take 2-3 tablespoons of red clay powder.

- Add a teaspoon of ground wheat germ and oatmeal.

- Add mineral water.

- Keep stirring until you get a sour cream-like density.

- Apply to the entire face, even around the eyes.

- Top it off with gauze soaked in warm water.

- Leave it on for 15-20 minutes.

- Remove with cosmetic wipes soaked in warm water.

- Dry your face and do not forget to use moisturizing cream at the end.

Body skincare

Clay promotes the restoration of natural skin functions while removing toxins, helping cell regeneration, and returning skin its healthy look.

Be sure to only use clay that matches your skin type: very soft white clay is recommended for irritable, thin, dry, and mature skin; red clay is great for oily, red, and very sensitive skin; yellow clay is suitable for skin that falls into numerous category types as well as for skin that is usually red and irritated.

Deep body cleaning

Do you wish to prepare yourself for the summer holidays? It is hard to find an easier way to improve your appearance in a short period of time than simply doing a deep cleaning of your entire body's skin:

- Add half of a pound of white clay into a glass.

- Add a tablespoon of lightly ground almonds and a tablespoon of seaweed crushed into powder.

- Stir well.

- Add warm water and orange blossom extract.

- Take a shower. During the shower gently wipe down your skin.

- Turn off the shower.

- Then while massaging almond crumbs into your skin spread the clay, which should have a consistency of sour cream, all over your body.

- Afterwards, wash off the mask with hot water while rubbing your skin.

Mask for the chest

This mask not only cleanses but also softens your skin giving you a sense of invigoration and a pleasant aroma to your body.

- Pour a quarter to a half of a pound of pink clay powder into a cup.

- Add mineral water.

- Add myrrh, rosemary, and lavender essential oils—a drop of each.

- Apply a thick mask on your breasts and leave it on for 20 minutes.

- Remove the majority of the mask with your hands.

- Remove the rest with soaked cosmetic wipes or a shower.

- Make up to 2 masks a week.

Softening bath

Hard water tends to irritate sensitive skin over time. Remedy the situation with a bath:

- Prepare an infusion, on the side, with bran and oatmeal—a handful of each per quart of water.

- Add approximately 10 drops of rosemary essential oil, a glass of olive oil, and red clay powder.

- Mix and pour into a bath.

- Bathe for 20 minutes and then rinse off with a shower.

- Apply body oil or moisturizing cream.

Relaxing bath

Our daily lives are filled with stress. A relaxing bath is a great way to let go, unwind, and improve your mood:

- Make a bath and add a small pack of pink clay powder.

- Prior to the bath, prepare a cold infusion with verbena, rosemary, and thyme.

- Pour it into a bath and add some drops of tangerine oil.

- Take a bath for about an hour, and then rinse off with a shower.

- Cover your body with moisturizing cream and enjoy a good night's rest.

Stimulating Bath

After a busy day or a tiresome party, take a stimulating bath to regain vitality and strength:

- Make a bath.

- Add 5-6 drops of rosemary essential oil.

- Add 10 drops of thyme oil and mint oil.

- Add a handful of seaweed crushed to powder.

- Add a half of a pound of yellow clay powder.

- The water should not be less than 100 °F.

- Submerge and enjoy for 20 minutes.

- Rinse off with a hot shower and enjoy your day.

Hair care

Depending on the length of your hair, you will require a different quantity of ingredients.

For long hair you may need as much as a half of a pound of clay while only a quarter pound of clay will suffice if you have short hair.

Mask for all types of hair

- Pour warm water, about 100 °F, into a glass.

- Add a teaspoon of lemon juice and a tablespoon of apple vinegar.

- Mix thoroughly.

- Then add clay powder and continue to mix until you have a sour cream-like consistency.

- Use a wide brush to brush a small quantity of hair at a time until you cover the entire area.

- Put on a shower cap. The cap will prevent the clay from running down your face as well as from drying up.

- Boil some water in a pot and keep a towel over it until it becomes soaked from the steam. Be careful not burn yourself.

- Place the towel on top of your shower cap; the heat will further activate clay.

- Keep the mask on for 20 minutes.

- Take off the towel and the shower cap.

- First remove as much clay as you can with your hands and then thoroughly wash off the rest with water.

- Afterwards, cleanse your scalp with a shampoo that has green clay in it.

- Then, apply a revitalizing conditioner to your hair.

Mask to combat hair loss

Prepare a mask to strengthen hair roots and to stimulate hair growth:

- Add 1/2-1 pound of white clay powder to a ceramic or glass bowl.

- Add 2-3 drops of rosemary essential oil and some warm water.

- Stir until you reach a homogeneous sour cream-like consistency.

- Apply to your scalp with the help of a brush.

- Leave it on for 20 minutes.

- Thoroughly wash your hair with warm water.

- Make this mask 2-3 times a week.

- Continue for 3-6 months.

Do not be alarmed if you notice an increase in hair loss while washing your hair after the first few masks. The hair strands falling out are the ones with damaged roots and would have fallen out eventually anyways.

Be patient, though. Continue to apply clay as it should help to activate your hair growth.

You can alternate between white and green clay. Carefully observe the effect throughout the process; in a few months your hair should return to normal showing its beauty and health once again.

Mask for oily, weak and damaged hair

It should not take you long to go from dandruff-ridden, oily hair to healthy, shiny hair when you prepare this mask:

- Get a clean cup.

- For long and short hair, add about a quarter of a pound of green clay powder.

- Add a teaspoon of apple vinegar.

- A few drops of sage essential oil.

- And squeeze one lemon into the cup.

- Apply a thick layer to your scalp.

- Leave it on for 15-20 minutes.

- Remove as much as you can with your hands and thoroughly wash off the rest with water.

- Then use moisturizing shampoo.

- Make this mask 2-3 times a week.

The first applications are especially important as clay works to regulate and revitalize your sebaceous glands. Subsequently, you can apply it less often because gradually your hair should gain enough volume and silkiness from one application to last you an entire week.

Mask for dry hair

Whatever your hair length, the preparation of this mask uses the same quantity of ingredients—just as with oily hair. Applications are made in the same way as well:

- Add white or pink clay powder to a cup.

- Add lemon juice.

- Add 1 drop of lavender essential oil.

- Add 10 drops of nutmeg oil.

- Stir and apply.

- On the side, boil a pot of water and place a towel over it so that it becomes hot and soaked with steam. Be careful not to burn the towel or yourself.

- Wrap your head with the soaked towel over the mask to further activate clay.

- Remove the towel and the mask after 15 minutes.

- Thoroughly wash off the clay, and then shampoo your hair and apply moisturizing conditioner.

Mask for thinning hair and hair with split ends

Thin, splitting, dry hair has a frightful, shameful appearance.

To work back to a healthy look, first, it is necessary to strengthen your hair:

- Consider the length of your hair when preparing this mask. Use a quarter to half of a pound of white or pink clay powder.

- Add a spoonful of avocado oil, a teaspoon of apple vinegar, and one egg yolk.

- Use a mixer for up to 5 minutes to blend it.

- It should be homogeneous, smooth, and not too dense so that you can easily spread it on your hair.

- Depending on your desired effect, apply a thin or a thick layer all over your scalp for up to 20 minutes.

- Remove as much as you can with your hands and thoroughly wash off the rest with water, and then use a shampoo for dry hair to wash your hair twice.

- Finish off with a moisturizing conditioner.

Very soon your hair will have a natural shine, strength, and elasticity that you were looking for.

Hand and foot care

Softening mask for hands

To have beautiful hands, you need to constantly care for them:

- Mix a little bit of olive oil with warm water.

- Pour into a bowl with clay and stir until you have a homogeneous sour cream-like consistency.

- Submerge your hands into the bowl that you used to prepare the mask.

- Place both hands into the mix for about 20 minutes, wash them off, and apply moisturizing cream while gently massaging your fingers, palms, and wrists to get more blood flow.

Bath for tired feet

After a long day on your feet, you can feel them start to pulsate and slightly shake. When you are home at last, you should immediately prepare a hot bath (in a small tub or tray) for your feet with a water temperature of about 100 °F:

- Add a handful of large grey salt, a few drops of mint oil, and lavender oil.

- Stir and add a handful of green clay powder.

- Now submerge your feet into the little bath of your creation.

- Make this bath whenever you need it.

Bath for swollen feet

Feet often swell as a result of poor blood circulation. Use a small clay bath to get you back on track:

- Prepare a small tub with warm water.

- Add handful of clay granules.

- Add a handful of seaweed crushed into powder and half of a handful of sea salt.

- As soon as the clay is dissolved, submerge your feet into the tub.

- Make this bath when you need it.

Bath for hurting feet

When your feet hurt, you can make simple little baths with clay powder, preferably with green clay:

- Pour warm water into a little tub.

- Add 2 handfuls of clay powder.

- Add 10 drops of juniper essential oil to relieve pain.

- Keep your feet submerged for about 20 minutes.

- Make this bath when you need it.

Clay Secrets

Bibliography

Antonova, Irina. Healing with Clay: Questions and Answers. Galeos, 2006.

Bereginia, Nina. Clay, the Natural Healer. CHAO, 1999.

Kochenko, Nadia. Medicinal Properties of Clay. Moscow: Astrel, 2001.

Milash, Mary. Healing Clay and Healing Mud. ACT Owl, 2006.

Petrov, Valera. Clay Minerals. <http://bse.sci-lib.com/article010931.html>. August 29, 2011.

Pokrovski, Boris. Let's Heal with Clay. 155 Best Recipes. ACC Lada Center, 2005.

Romanova, Olga. Cleansing Through Natural Means. Vector, 2009.

Semyonava, Hope. Age reversing and healing with Clay. Dealia, 2007.

Shuvalova, Olga. Healing with clay and mud. Nevski Prospect, 2000.

Sokolov, Vacheslav. Types of clay and its characteristics. <http://www.pereplet.ru/obrazovanie/stsoros/1073.html>. September 3, 2011.

Sokolava, Tatiana and Tatiana Dronava. Clay Minerals in the Ground. Toola, 2005.

Travinka, Valentina. Blue Healing Clay. St. Petersburg: St. Petersburg Press, 2000.

95

Clay Secrets

About the Author

Born and raised in Soviet Russia, Matt Isaac emigrated from St. Petersburg, Russia to Cleveland, Ohio shortly after the collapse of the Berlin Wall. Ever since his immigration, he found himself fascinated with the different approaches to medicine between his old country and new. He is now fully dedicated to examining modern health solutions with a cultural twist.

www.ingramcontent.com/pod-product-compliance
Lightning Source LLC
Chambersburg PA
CBHW050538280326
41933CB00011B/1638